Welcome to MedWise Scholar – your compass for navigating the world of pharmacy and healthcare. Congratulations on taking the first step with this study guide, designed to elevate your understanding of medications and enhance your healthcare journey.

As you delve into its insights, consider exploring our range of study aides, thoughtfully curated to bolster your learning experience. MedWise Scholar is here to empower your success every step of the way.

We appreciate your trust in us as your educational partner, and we're excited to join you on this path to professional excellence. Thank you for choosing MedWise Scholar!

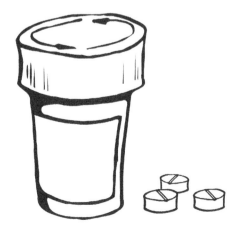

DRUG SUFFIXES

DRUG SUFFIX	EXAMPLES	INDICATION	DEFINITION
–azepam	lorazepam	Anxiety, Insomnia	Antianxiety agents (diazepam type)
–pred–	prednicarbate, cloprednol	Arthritis, Asthma	Prednisone derivatives
–terol	albuterol	Asthma	(phenethylamine derivatives)
–bactam	sulbactam	Bacterial Infections	Beta–lactamase inhibitors
cef–	cefazolin	Bacterial Infections	Cephalosporins (first-gen)
–cillin	oxacillin	Bacterial Infections	Penicillins
–cycline	tetracycline	Bacterial Infections	Antibiotics (tetracycline type)
–mycin	lincomycin	Bacterial Infections	Antibiotics (streptomyces strains)
–sulfa	sulfasalazine	Bacterial Infections	Antibiotics (sulfonamide derivatives)
–oxetine	duloxetine	Depression	Antidepressants
–pramine	lofepramine	Depression	Antidepressants (imipramine type)
–triptyline	amitriptyline	Depression	Antidepressants
–gliptin	vildagliptin	Diabetes Mellitus	Antihyperglycemics
–afil	sildenafil	Erectile Dysfunction	Inhibitor of PDE5 with vasodilator action
–etanide	bumetanide	Fluid Retention	Diuretics
–conazole	fluconazole	Fungal Infections	Antifungals (miconazole type)
–prazole	omeprazole	GERD, Erosive Esophagitis	Proton-pump inhibitor

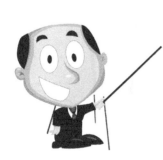

Learning these drug suffixes will assist you in learning your drug list.

DRUG SUFFIX	EXAMPLES		
–prost–	latanoprost, unoprostone	G	e
–fibrate	bezafibrate	H	
–statin	pepstatin	H. Hypercholesterol emia	inhibitor pepsin inhibitor
–alol	labetalol	Hypertension	Combined alpha and beta blockers
–azosin	doxazosin	Hypertension	Antihypertensives (prazosin type)
–olol	timolol	Hypertension	Beta–blockers (propranolol type)
–pamide	adipamide	Hypertension	Diuretics (sulfamoylbenzoic acid derivatives)
–pril	captopril	Hypertension	Antihypertensives (ACE inhibitors)
–sartan	losartan	Hypertension	Angiotensin II receptor antagonists
–pamil	tiapamil	Irregular Heart beat	Coronary vasodilators
–imus	napirimus	Organ Transplant	Immunosuppresives
–dronate	etidronate	Osteoprosis	Calcium metabolism regulators
–profen	flurbiprofen	Pain	Anti–inflammatory/an algesic agents (ibuprofen type)
–caine	lidocaine	Pain	Local anesthetics
–giline	selegiline	disease	MAO-inhibitors, type B
–grel–	ticagrelor	prevent stroke, heart attack, and other heart problems.	Platelet aggregation inhibitor
–fenamic acid	mefenamic acid	Rheumatoid diseases	Anti-inflammatory agents
–peridol	haloperidol	Schizophrenia	Antipsychotics (haloperidol type)
–peridone	iloperidone	Schizophrenia	Antispsychotics (risperidone type)
–barb–	phenobarbital	Seizures, Epilepsy	Barbituric acid derivatives
–glitazar	farglitazar	Type 2 Diabetes	Antihyperglycemics, PPRA agonists
–glizatone	rosiglitazone	Type 2 Diabetes	Antihyperglycemics, PPST agonists
–tide	Octreotide	Type 2 Diabetes	peptides and glycopeptides
vir-, -vir- or -vir	viroxime	Viral Infections	Antiviral substances (undefined group)

3

Notes

Welcome to this section of the study guide, tailored to help you master the TOP 200 Drugs with ease, just like using flash cards!

Here's how to make the most of this guide

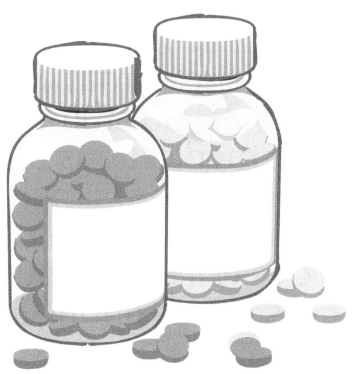

MASTERING BRAND & GENERIC NAMES

On the first page, you'll find the brand name of a medication. Flip to the next page to confirm your grasp of the associated generic drug name and the purpose of the medication.

Under each drug, you'll notice circles that come in handy. If you stumble upon medications that challenge you, simply mark them. These marked circles will act as your focus points during later reviews.

3 Ways to Optimize Your Learning:

Front-to-Back Review: Start by going through the list in order, reinforcing your knowledge of generic medications.

Back-to-Front Review: Next, switch it up and review from the end to the beginning. This helps you solidify your understanding of brand medications.

Random Page Challenge:
Once you're feeling confident with the list, add some fun unpredictability. Open the guide to random pages and put your knowledge to the test.

As you journey through these learning phases, rely on the circles you've marked. They'll guide you to the medications that need a little extra attention.

Remember, learning is a process, and this guide is your personalized roadmap to success. Happy studying!

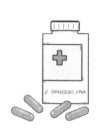

Brand

Provigil

PASS/FAIL

○○○○○○○○○○

Concerta

PASS/FAIL

○○○○○○○○○○

GENERIC

Modafinil

ADHD

PASS/FAIL

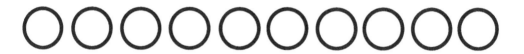

Methylphenidate

ADHD

PASS/FAIL

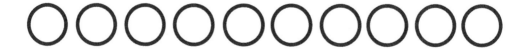

Brand

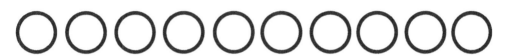

Vyvanse

PASS/FAIL

○○○○○○○○○○

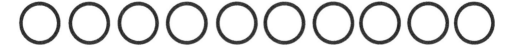

Focalin

PASS/FAIL

○○○○○○○○○○

GENERIC

Lisdexamfetamine

ADHD

PASS/FAIL

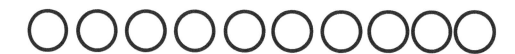

Dexmethylphenidate

ADHD

PASS/FAIL

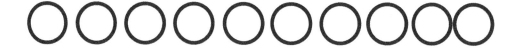

Brand

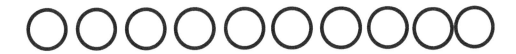

Strattera

PASS/FAIL

○○○○○○○○○○

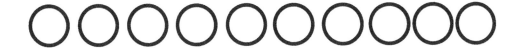

Adderall

PASS/FAIL

○○○○○○○○○○

GENERIC

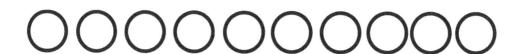

Atomoxetine

ADHD

PASS/FAIL

○○○○○○○○○○

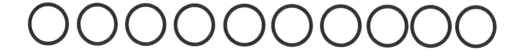

**Amphetamine /
Dextroamphetamine**

ADHD

PASS/FAIL

○○○○○○○○○○

Brand

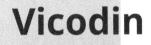

Vicodin

PASS/FAIL

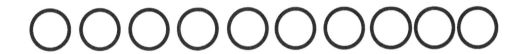

Ultram

PASS/FAIL

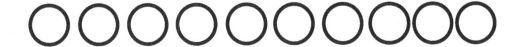

GENERIC

Hydrocodone/APAP

Analgesic

PASS/FAIL

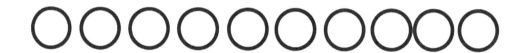

Tramadol

Class

PASS/FAIL

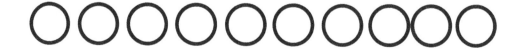

Brand

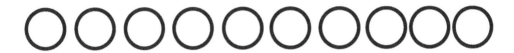

PASS/FAIL

OOOOOOOOOO

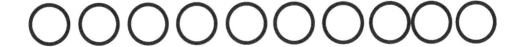

PASS/FAIL

OOOOOOOOOO

GENERIC

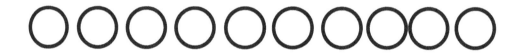

Oxycodone/APAP

Analgesic

PASS/FAIL

○○○○○○○○○○

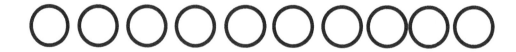

Oxycodone

Analgesic

PASS/FAIL

○○○○○○○○○○

Brand

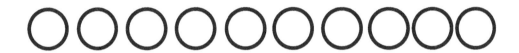

Tylenol #3

PASS/FAIL

◯◯◯◯◯◯◯◯◯◯

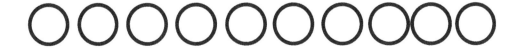

Duragesic

PASS/FAIL

◯◯◯◯◯◯◯◯◯◯

GENERIC

Codeine / APAP

Analgesic

PASS/FAIL

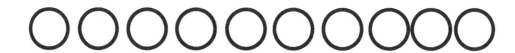

Fentanyl

Analgesic

PASS/FAIL

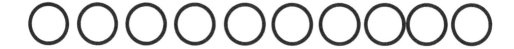

Brand

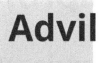

PASS/FAIL

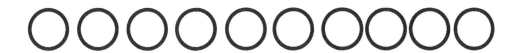

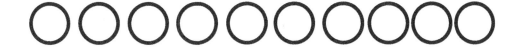

Mobic

PASS/FAIL

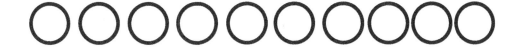

21

GENERIC

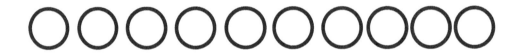

Ibuprofen

Analgesic (NSAID)

PASS/FAIL

○○○○○○○○○○

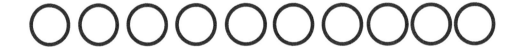

Meloxicam

Analgesic (NSAID)

PASS/FAIL

○○○○○○○○○○

Brand

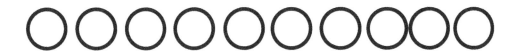

Celebrex

PASS/FAIL

OOOOOOOOOO

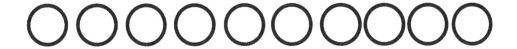

Aleve

PASS/FAIL

OOOOOOOOOO

GENERIC

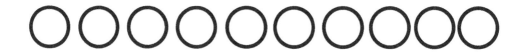

Celecoxib

Analgesic (NSAID)

PASS/FAIL

○○○○○○○○○○

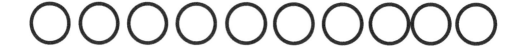

Naproxen

Analgesic (NSAID)

PASS/FAIL

○○○○○○○○○○

Brand

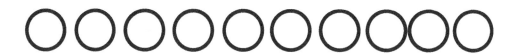

PASS/FAIL

◯◯◯◯◯◯◯◯◯◯

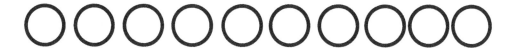

PASS/FAIL

◯◯◯◯◯◯◯◯◯◯

GENERIC

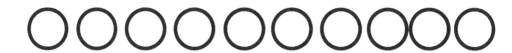

Nabumetone

Analgesic (NSAID)

PASS/FAIL

○○○○○○○○○○

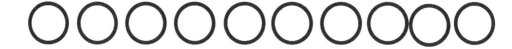

Diclofenac

Analgesic (NSAID)

PASS/FAIL

○○○○○○○○○○

Brand

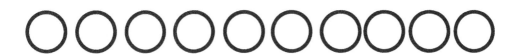

Pyridium

PASS/FAIL

○○○○○○○○○○

Zantac

PASS/FAIL

○○○○○○○○○○

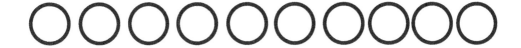

GENERIC

Phenazopyridine

Analgesic (urinary)

PASS/FAIL

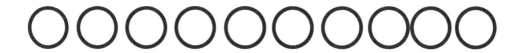

Ranitidine

Antacid (H2)

PASS/FAIL

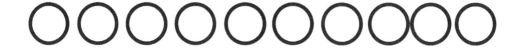

Brand

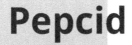

Pepcid

PASS/FAIL

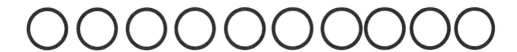

Nexium

PASS/FAIL

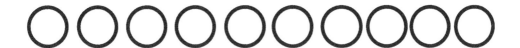

GENERIC

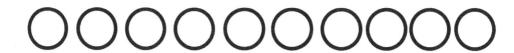

Famotidine

Antacid (H2)

PASS/FAIL

○○○○○○○○○○

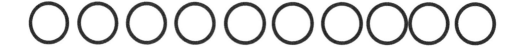

Esomeprazole

Class

PASS/FAIL

○○○○○○○○○○

Brand

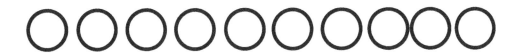

Prilosec

PASS/FAIL

◯◯◯◯◯◯◯◯◯◯

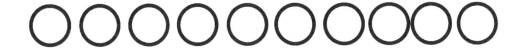

Protonix

PASS/FAIL

◯◯◯◯◯◯◯◯◯◯

GENERIC

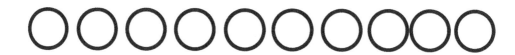

Omeprazole

Antacid (PPI)

PASS/FAIL

○○○○○○○○○○

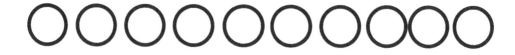

Pantoprazole

Antacid (PPI)

PASS/FAIL

○○○○○○○○○○

Brand

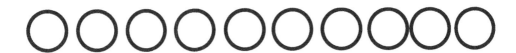

Dexilant

PASS/FAIL

○○○○○○○○○○

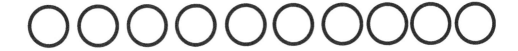

Aciphex

PASS/FAIL

○○○○○○○○○○

GENERIC

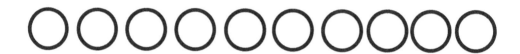

Dexlansoprazole

Antacid (PPI)

PASS/FAIL

○○○○○○○○○○

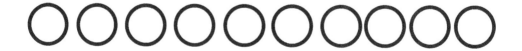

Rabeprazole

Antacid (PPI)

PASS/FAIL

○○○○○○○○○○

Brand

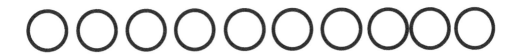

Prevacid

PASS/FAIL

○○○○○○○○○○

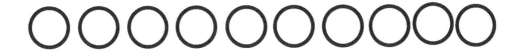

NitroStat SL

PASS/FAIL

○○○○○○○○○○

GENERIC

Lansoprazole

Antacid (PPI)

PASS/FAIL

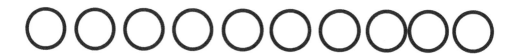

Nitroglycerine

Anti-angina

PASS/FAIL

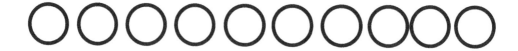

Brand

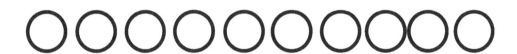

Enbrel

PASS/FAIL

○○○○○○○○○○

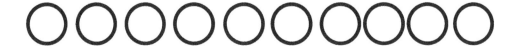

Singulair

PASS/FAIL

○○○○○○○○○○

GENERIC

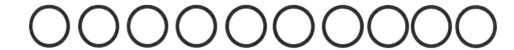

Etanercept

Anti-arthritic

PASS/FAIL

OOOOOOOOOO

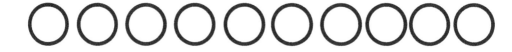

Montelukast

Anti-asthmatic

PASS/FAIL

OOOOOOOOOO

Brand

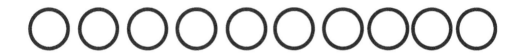

ProAir HFA

PASS/FAIL

○○○○○○○○○○

Uceris

PASS/FAIL

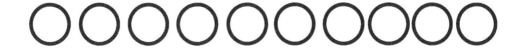

○○○○○○○○○○

39

GENERIC

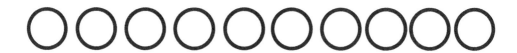

Albuterol

Anti-asthmatic

PASS/FAIL

○○○○○○○○○○

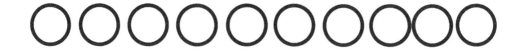

Budesonide

Anti-inflammatory

PASS/FAIL

○○○○○○○○○○

Brand

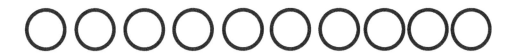

Medrol

PASS/FAIL

◯◯◯◯◯◯◯◯◯◯

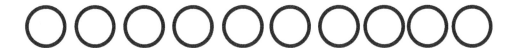

Deltasone

PASS/FAIL

◯◯◯◯◯◯◯◯◯◯

GENERIC

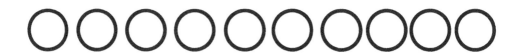

Methylprednisolone

Anti-inflammatory steriod

PASS/FAIL

○○○○○○○○○○

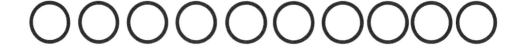

Prednisone

Anti-inflammatory steriod

PASS/FAIL

○○○○○○○○○○

Brand

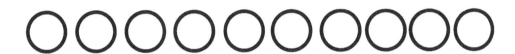

Clovate

PASS/FAIL

○○○○○○○○○○

Kenalog

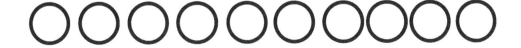

PASS/FAIL

○○○○○○○○○○

GENERIC

Clobetasol

Anti-inflammatory steriod

PASS/FAIL

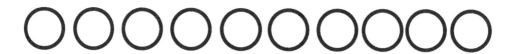

Triamcinolone

Anti-inflammatory steriod

PASS/FAIL

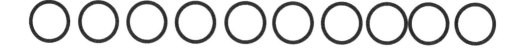

44

Brand

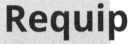

Requip

PASS/FAIL

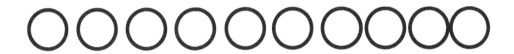

Cogentin

PASS/FAIL

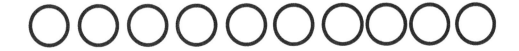

GENERIC

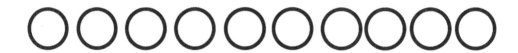

Ropinirole

Anti-Parkinson's

PASS/FAIL

○○○○○○○○○○

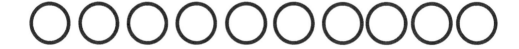

Benztropine

Anti-Parkinson's

PASS/FAIL

○○○○○○○○○○

Brand

Mirapex

PASS/FAIL

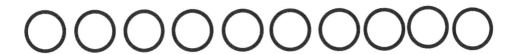

Sinemet

PASS/FAIL

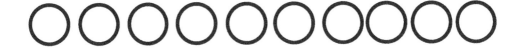

GENERIC

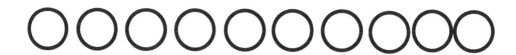

Pramipexole

Anti-Parkinson's

PASS/FAIL

◯◯◯◯◯◯◯◯◯◯

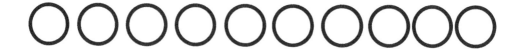

Levodopa

Anti-Parkinson's

PASS/FAIL

◯◯◯◯◯◯◯◯◯◯

Brand

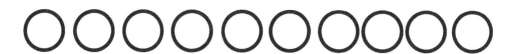

Stalevo 50

PASS/FAIL

○○○○○○○○○○

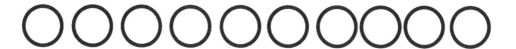

Chantix

PASS/FAIL

○○○○○○○○○○

GENERIC

Carbidopa / Levodopa / Entacapone

Anti-Parkinson's

PASS/FAIL

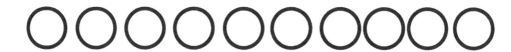

Varenicline

Anti-smoking

PASS/FAIL

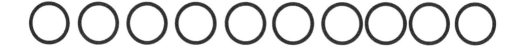

Brand

Xanax

PASS/FAIL

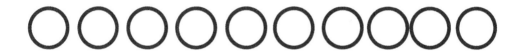

Klonopin

PASS/FAIL

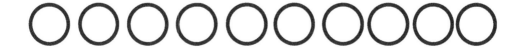

GENERIC

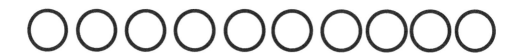

Alprazolam

Antianxiety

PASS/FAIL

◯◯◯◯◯◯◯◯◯◯

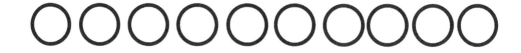

Clonazepam

Antianxiety

PASS/FAIL

◯◯◯◯◯◯◯◯◯◯

Brand

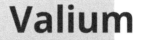

PASS/FAIL

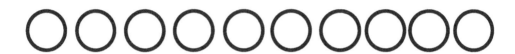

OOOOOOOOOO

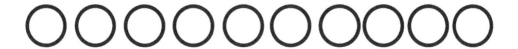

PASS/FAIL

OOOOOOOOOO

GENERIC

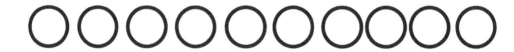

Diazepam

Antianxiety

PASS/FAIL

○○○○○○○○○○

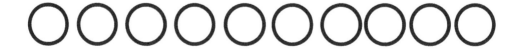

Lorazepam

Antianxiety

PASS/FAIL

○○○○○○○○○○

Brand

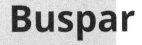

PASS/FAIL

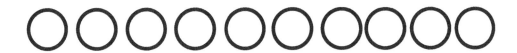

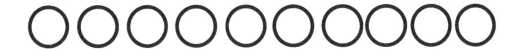

PASS/FAIL

GENERIC

Buspirone

Antianxiety

PASS/FAIL

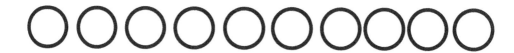

Amoxicillin

Antibiotic

PASS/FAIL

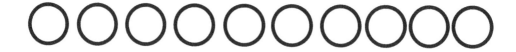

Brand

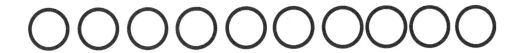

Zithromax

PASS/FAIL

○○○○○○○○○○

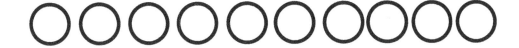

Keflex

PASS/FAIL

○○○○○○○○○○

GENERIC

Azithromycin

Antibiotic

PASS/FAIL

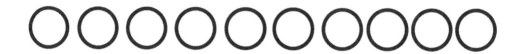

Cephalexin

Antibiotic

PASS/FAIL

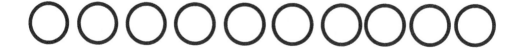

Brand

Vibramycin

PASS/FAIL

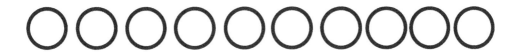

Levaquin

PASS/FAIL

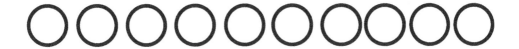

GENERIC

Doxycycline

Antibiotic

PASS/FAIL

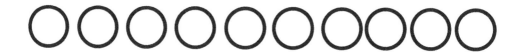

Levofloxacin

Antibiotic

PASS/FAIL

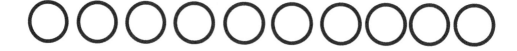

Brand

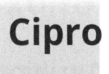

PASS/FAIL

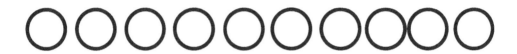

Pen VK

PASS/FAIL

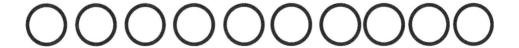

GENERIC

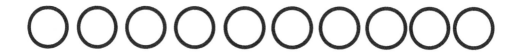

Ciprofloxacin

Antibiotic

PASS/FAIL

○○○○○○○○○○

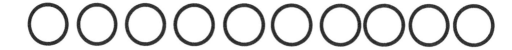

Penicillin

Antibiotic

PASS/FAIL

○○○○○○○○○○

Brand

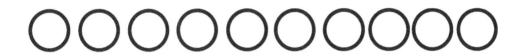

Omnicef

PASS/FAIL

◯◯◯◯◯◯◯◯◯◯

Cleocin

PASS/FAIL

◯◯◯◯◯◯◯◯◯◯

GENERIC

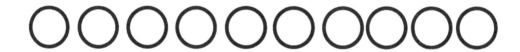

Cefdinir

Antibiotic

PASS/FAIL

○○○○○○○○○○

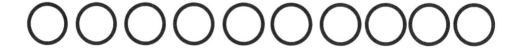

Clindamycin

Antibiotic

PASS/FAIL

○○○○○○○○○○

Brand

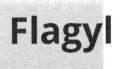

PASS/FAIL

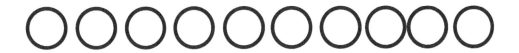

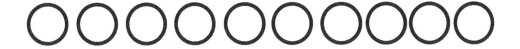

PASS/FAIL

GENERIC

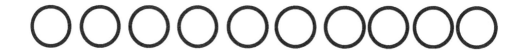

Metronidazole

Antibiotic

PASS/FAIL

◯◯◯◯◯◯◯◯◯◯

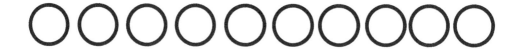

Moxifloxacin

Antibiotic

PASS/FAIL

◯◯◯◯◯◯◯◯◯◯

Brand

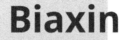

PASS/FAIL

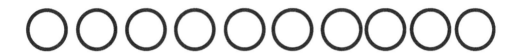

Minocin

PASS/FAIL

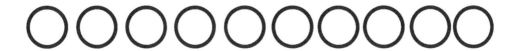

GENERIC

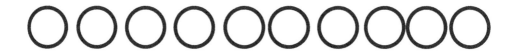

Clarithromycin

Antibiotic

PASS/FAIL

○○○○○○○○○○

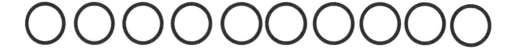

Minocycline

Antibiotic

PASS/FAIL

○○○○○○○○○○

Brand

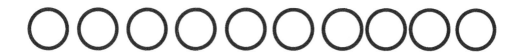

Macrobid

PASS/FAIL

○○○○○○○○○○

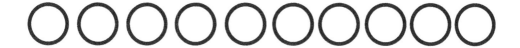

Ceftin

PASS/FAIL

○○○○○○○○○○

GENERIC

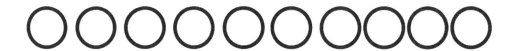

Nitrofurantoin

Antibiotic

PASS/FAIL

◯◯◯◯◯◯◯◯◯◯

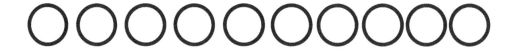

Cefuroxime

Antibiotic

PASS/FAIL

◯◯◯◯◯◯◯◯◯◯

Brand

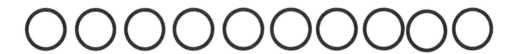

Bactroban

PASS/FAIL

○○○○○○○○○○

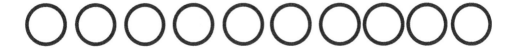

Plavix

PASS/FAIL

○○○○○○○○○○

GENERIC

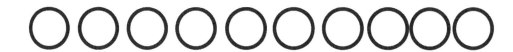

Mupirocin

Antibiotic

PASS/FAIL

○○○○○○○○○○

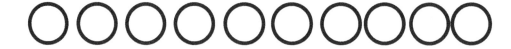

Clopidogrel

Anticoagulant

PASS/FAIL

○○○○○○○○○○

Brand

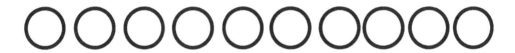

Coumadin

PASS/FAIL

○○○○○○○○○○

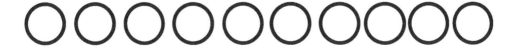

Xarelto

PASS/FAIL

○○○○○○○○○○

GENERIC

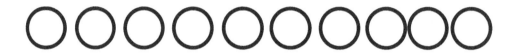

Warfarin

Anticoagulant

PASS/FAIL

○○○○○○○○○○

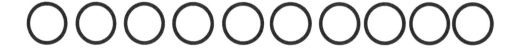

Rivaroxaban

Anticoagulant

PASS/FAIL

○○○○○○○○○○

74

Brand

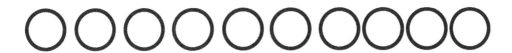

Lovenox

PASS/FAIL

○○○○○○○○○○

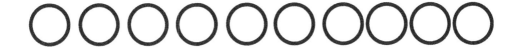

Pradaxa

PASS/FAIL

○○○○○○○○○○

GENERIC

Enoxaparin

Anticoagulant

PASS/FAIL

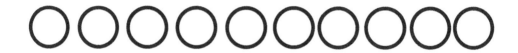

Dabigatran

Class

PASS/FAIL

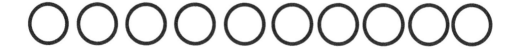

Brand

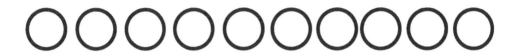

Ticagrelor

PASS/FAIL

○○○○○○○○○○

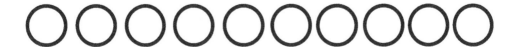

Neurontin

PASS/FAIL

○○○○○○○○○○

GENERIC

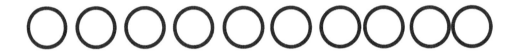

Brilinta

Anticoagulant

PASS/FAIL

○○○○○○○○○○

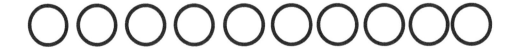

Gabapentin

Anticonvulsant

PASS/FAIL

○○○○○○○○○○

Brand

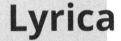

PASS/FAIL

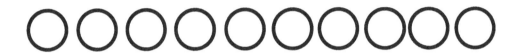

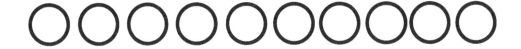

PASS/FAIL

○○○○○○○○○○

GENERIC

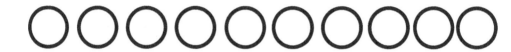

Pregabalin

Anticonvulsant

PASS/FAIL

○○○○○○○○○○

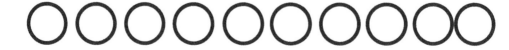

Topiramate

Anticonvulsant

PASS/FAIL

○○○○○○○○○○

Brand

Depakote

PASS/FAIL

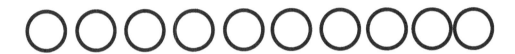

Dilantin

PASS/FAIL

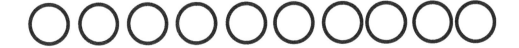

GENERIC

Divalproex

Anticonvulsant

PASS/FAIL

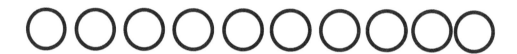

Phenytoin

Anticonvulsant

PASS/FAIL

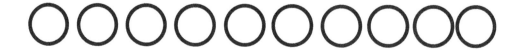

Brand

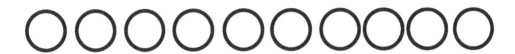

Namenda

PASS/FAIL

○○○○○○○○○○

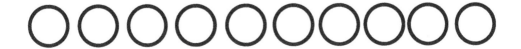

Exelon

PASS/FAIL

○○○○○○○○○○

GENERIC

Memantine

Antidementia

PASS/FAIL

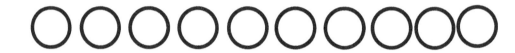

Rivastigmine

Antidementia

PASS/FAIL

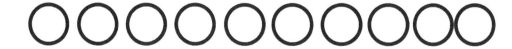

Brand

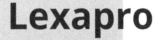

Lexapro

PASS/FAIL

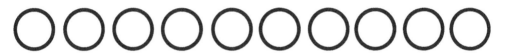

Zoloft

PASS/FAIL

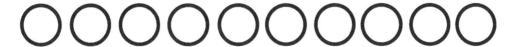

GENERIC

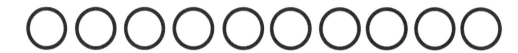

Escitalopram

Antidepressant

PASS/FAIL

○○○○○○○○○○

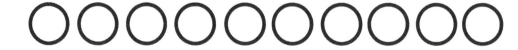

Sertraline

Antidepressant

PASS/FAIL

○○○○○○○○○○

Brand

Desyrel

PASS/FAIL

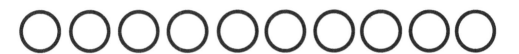

Cymbalta

PASS/FAIL

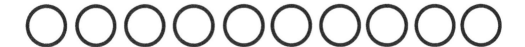

GENERIC

Trazodone

Antidepressant

PASS/FAIL

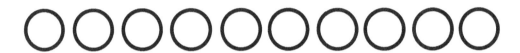

Duloxetine

Antidepressant

PASS/FAIL

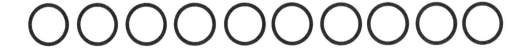

Brand

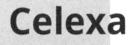

PASS/FAIL

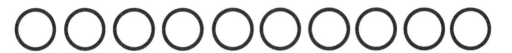

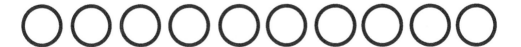

PASS/FAIL

○○○○○○○○○○

GENERIC

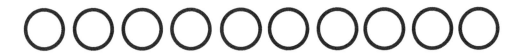

Citalopram

Antidepressant

PASS/FAIL

○○○○○○○○○○

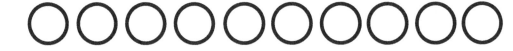

Paroxetine

Antidepressant

PASS/FAIL

○○○○○○○○○○

Brand

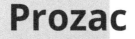

PASS/FAIL

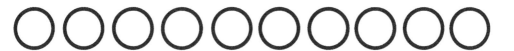

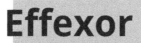

PASS/FAIL

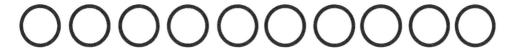

GENERIC

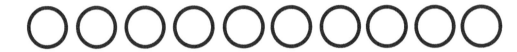

Fluoxetine

Antidepressant

PASS/FAIL

○○○○○○○○○○

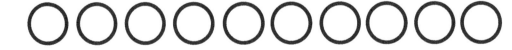

Venlafaxine

Antidepressant

PASS/FAIL

○○○○○○○○○○

Brand

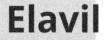

Elavil

PASS/FAIL

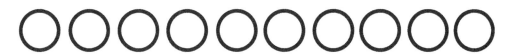

Wellbutrin

PASS/FAIL

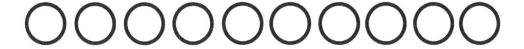

GENERIC

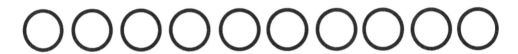

Amitriptyline

Antidepressant

PASS/FAIL

◯◯◯◯◯◯◯◯◯◯

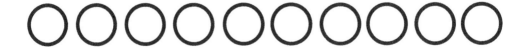

Bupropion

Antidepressant

PASS/FAIL

◯◯◯◯◯◯◯◯◯◯

Brand

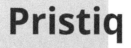

PASS/FAIL

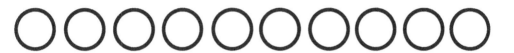

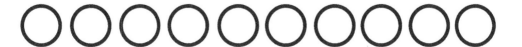

PASS/FAIL

○○○○○○○○○○

GENERIC

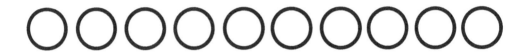

Desvenlafaxine

Antidepressant

PASS/FAIL

○○○○○○○○○○

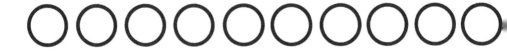

Nortriptyline

Antidepressant

PASS/FAIL

○○○○○○○○○○

Brand

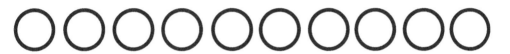

Remeron

PASS/FAIL

○○○○○○○○○○

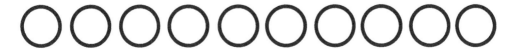

Glucophage

PASS/FAIL

○○○○○○○○○○

GENERIC

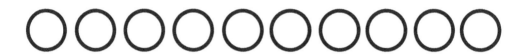

Mirtazepine

Antidepressant

PASS/FAIL

○○○○○○○○○○

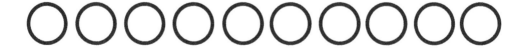

Metformin

Antidiabetic

PASS/FAIL

○○○○○○○○○○

Brand

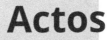

Actos

PASS/FAIL

○ ○ ○ ○ ○ ○ ○ ○ ○ ○

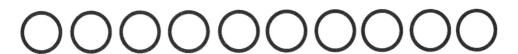

Levemir

PASS/FAIL

○ ○ ○ ○ ○ ○ ○ ○ ○ ○

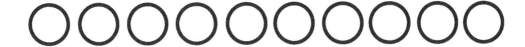

GENERIC

Pioglitazone

Antidiabetic

PASS/FAIL

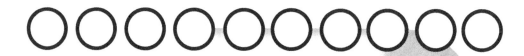

Insulin Detemir

Antidiabetic

PASS/FAIL

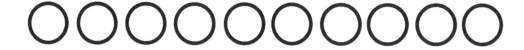

Brand

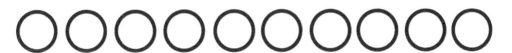

Novolog

PASS/FAIL

○○○○○○○○○○

Januvia

PASS/FAIL

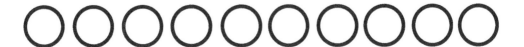

○○○○○○○○○○

GENERIC

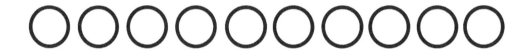

Insulin Aspart

Antidiabetic

PASS/FAIL

○ ○ ○ ○ ○ ○ ○ ○ ○ ○

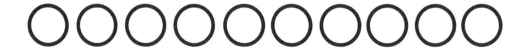

Sitagliptin

Antidiabetic

PASS/FAIL

○ ○ ○ ○ ○ ○ ○ ○ ○ ○

Brand

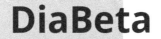

DiaBeta

PASS/FAIL

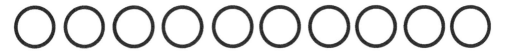

○○○○○○○○○○

Lantus

PASS/FAIL

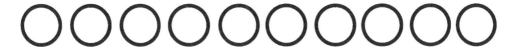

○○○○○○○○○○

GENERIC

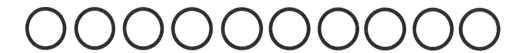

Glyburide

Antidiabetic

PASS/FAIL

○○○○○○○○○○

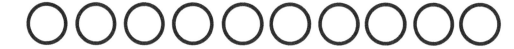

Insulin Glargine

Antidiabetic

PASS/FAIL

○○○○○○○○○○

Brand

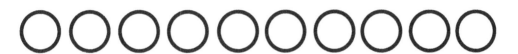

Glucotrol

PASS/FAIL

◯◯◯◯◯◯◯◯◯◯

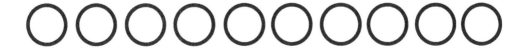

Humalog

PASS/FAIL

◯◯◯◯◯◯◯◯◯◯

GENERIC

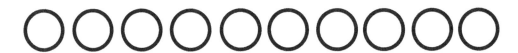

Glipizide

Antidiabetic

PASS/FAIL

○○○○○○○○○○

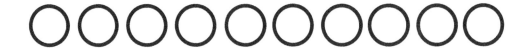

Insulin Lispro

Antidiabetic

PASS/FAIL

○○○○○○○○○○

Brand

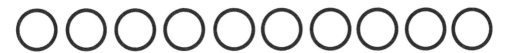

Victoza

PASS/FAIL

○○○○○○○○○○

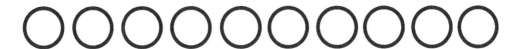

Onglyza

PASS/FAIL

○○○○○○○○○○

GENERIC

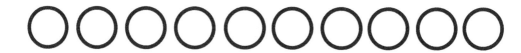

Liraglutide

Antidiabetic

PASS/FAIL

○○○○○○○○○○

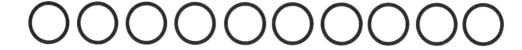

Saxagliptin

Antidiabetic

PASS/FAIL

○○○○○○○○○○

Brand

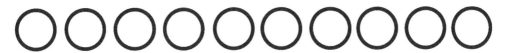

Dramamine

PASS/FAIL

○○○○○○○○○○

Zofran

PASS/FAIL

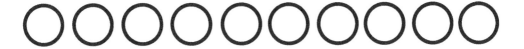

○○○○○○○○○○

GENERIC

Meclizine

Antiemetic

PASS/FAIL

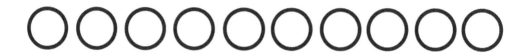

Ondansetron

Antiemetic

PASS/FAIL

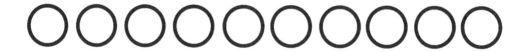

Brand

Lamictal

PASS/FAIL

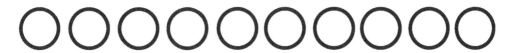

Diflucan

PASS/FAIL

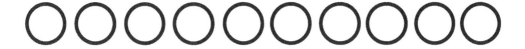

GENERIC

Lamotrigine

Antiepileptic

PASS/FAIL

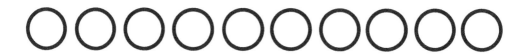

Fluconazole

Antifungal

PASS/FAIL

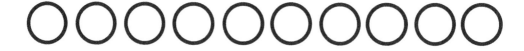

Brand

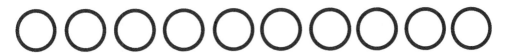

Nizoral

PASS/FAIL

◯◯◯◯◯◯◯◯◯◯

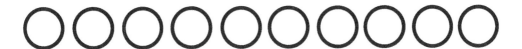

Lotrimin

PASS/FAIL

◯◯◯◯◯◯◯◯◯◯

GENERIC

Ketoconazole

Antifungal

PASS/FAIL

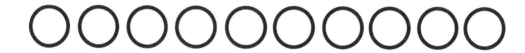

Clotrimazole

Antifungal

PASS/FAIL

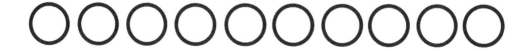

Brand

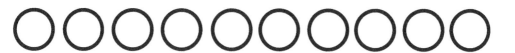

Xalatan

PASS/FAIL

○○○○○○○○○○

Travatan

PASS/FAIL

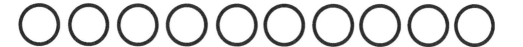

○○○○○○○○○○

GENERIC

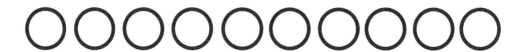

Latanoprost

Antiglaucoma

PASS/FAIL

○○○○○○○○○○

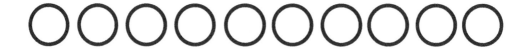

Travoprost

Antiglaucoma

PASS/FAIL

○○○○○○○○○○

Brand

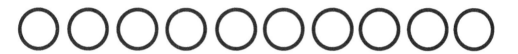

Zyloprim

PASS/FAIL

○○○○○○○○○○

Colcrys

PASS/FAIL

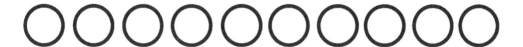

○○○○○○○○○○

GENERIC

Allopurinol

Antigout

PASS/FAIL

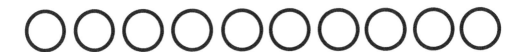

Colchicine

Antigout

PASS/FAIL

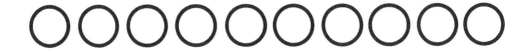

Brand

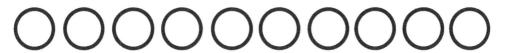

Uloric

PASS/FAIL

○○○○○○○○○○

Phenergan

PASS/FAIL

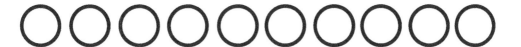

○○○○○○○○○○

GENERIC

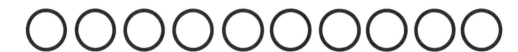

Febuxostat

Antigout

PASS/FAIL

◯◯◯◯◯◯◯◯◯◯

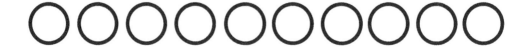

Promethazine

Antihistamine

PASS/FAIL

◯◯◯◯◯◯◯◯◯◯

Brand

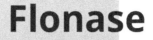

Flonase

PASS/FAIL

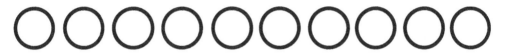

Allegra

PASS/FAIL

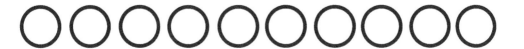

GENERIC

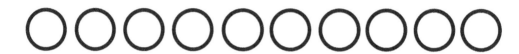

Fluticasone

Antihistamine

PASS/FAIL

○○○○○○○○○○

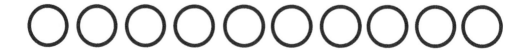

Fexofenadine

Antihistamine

PASS/FAIL

○○○○○○○○○○

Brand

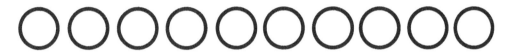

Nasonex

PASS/FAIL

◯◯◯◯◯◯◯◯◯◯

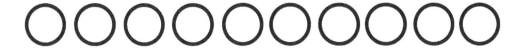

Zyrtec

PASS/FAIL

◯◯◯◯◯◯◯◯◯◯

GENERIC

Mometasone

Antihistamine

PASS/FAIL

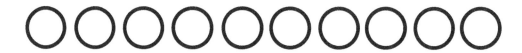

Cetirizine

Antihistamine

PASS/FAIL

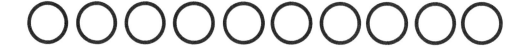

Brand

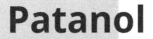

Patanol

PASS/FAIL

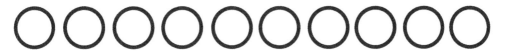

Prinivil

PASS/FAIL

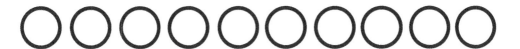

GENERIC

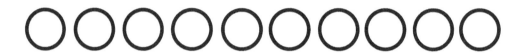

Olopatadine

Antihistamine

PASS/FAIL

○○○○○○○○○○

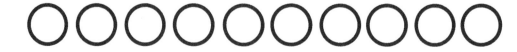

Lisinopril

Antihypertensive

PASS/FAIL

○○○○○○○○○○

Brand

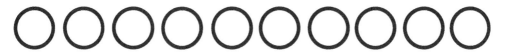

Lopressor

PASS/FAIL

○○○○○○○○○○

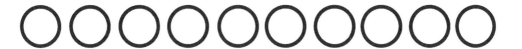

Diovan

PASS/FAIL

○○○○○○○○○○

GENERIC

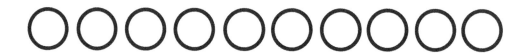

Metoprolol

Antihypertensive

PASS/FAIL

○○○○○○○○○○

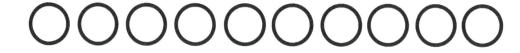

Valsartan

Antihypertensive

PASS/FAIL

○○○○○○○○○○

Brand

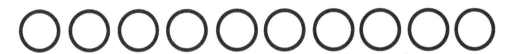

Norvasc

PASS/FAIL

○ ○ ○ ○ ○ ○ ○ ○ ○ ○

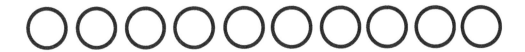

Lotensin

PASS/FAIL

○ ○ ○ ○ ○ ○ ○ ○ ○ ○

GENERIC

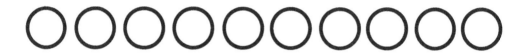

Amlodipine

Antihypertensive

PASS/FAIL

○○○○○○○○○○

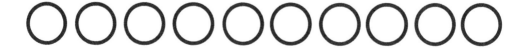

Benazepril

Antihypertensive

PASS/FAIL

○○○○○○○○○○

Brand

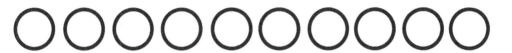

Coreg

PASS/FAIL

○○○○○○○○○○

Tenormin

PASS/FAIL

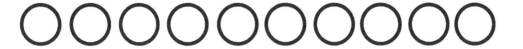

○○○○○○○○○○

GENERIC

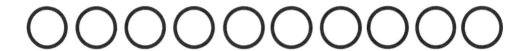

Carvedilol

Antihypertensive

PASS/FAIL

○○○○○○○○○○

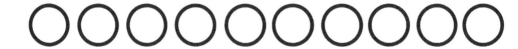

Atenolol

Antihypertensive

PASS/FAIL

○○○○○○○○○○

Brand

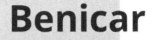

PASS/FAIL

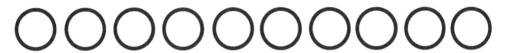

○○○○○○○○○○

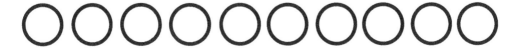

PASS/FAIL

○○○○○○○○○○

GENERIC

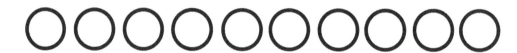

Olmesartan

Antihypertensive

PASS/FAIL

○○○○○○○○○○

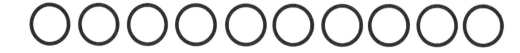

Enalapril

Antihypertensive

PASS/FAIL

○○○○○○○○○○

Brand

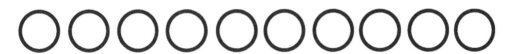

Catapres

PASS/FAIL

○○○○○○○○○○

Cardizem

PASS/FAIL

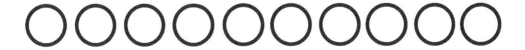

○○○○○○○○○○

GENERIC

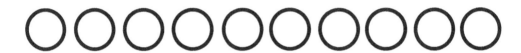

Clonidine

Antihypertensive

PASS/FAIL

○○○○○○○○○○

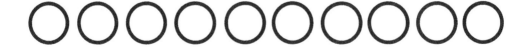

Diltiazem

Antihypertensive

PASS/FAIL

○○○○○○○○○○

Brand

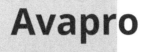

PASS/FAIL

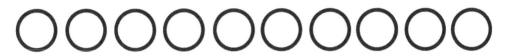

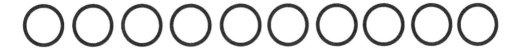

PASS/FAIL

GENERIC

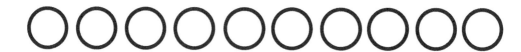

Irbesartan

Antihypertensive

PASS/FAIL

○○○○○○○○○○

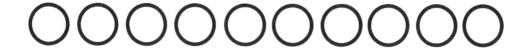

Losartan

Antihypertensive

PASS/FAIL

○○○○○○○○○○

Brand

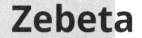

PASS/FAIL

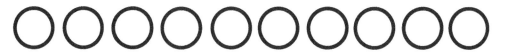

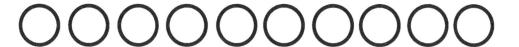

PASS/FAIL

GENERIC

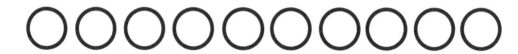

Bisoprolol

Antihypertensive

PASS/FAIL

○○○○○○○○○○

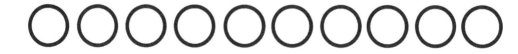

Ramipril

Antihypertensive

PASS/FAIL

○○○○○○○○○○

Brand

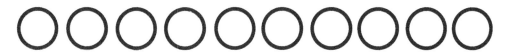

Accupril

PASS/FAIL

○ ○ ○ ○ ○ ○ ○ ○ ○ ○

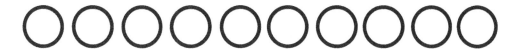

Proscar

PASS/FAIL

○ ○ ○ ○ ○ ○ ○ ○ ○ ○

GENERIC

Quinapril

Antihypertensive

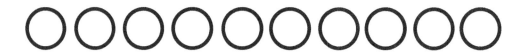

PASS/FAIL

○○○○○○○○○○

Finasteride

Antihypertensive

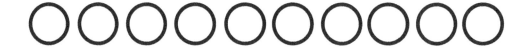

PASS/FAIL

○○○○○○○○○○

Brand

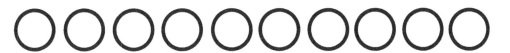

Avodart

PASS/FAIL

○○○○○○○○○○

Bystolic

PASS/FAIL

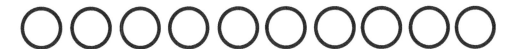

○○○○○○○○○○

GENERIC

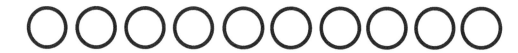

Dutasteride

Antihypertensive

PASS/FAIL

○○○○○○○○○○

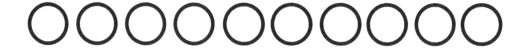

Nebivolol

Antihypertensive

PASS/FAIL

○○○○○○○○○○

Brand

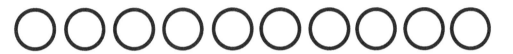

Procardia

PASS/FAIL

○○○○○○○○○○

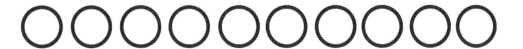

Hytrin

PASS/FAIL

○○○○○○○○○○

GENERIC

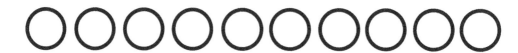

Nifedipine

Antihypertensive

PASS/FAIL

○○○○○○○○○○

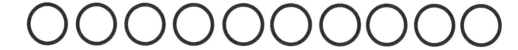

Terazosin

Antihypertensive

PASS/FAIL

○○○○○○○○○○

Brand

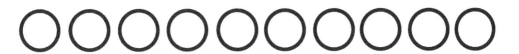

Apresoline

PASS/FAIL

○○○○○○○○○○

Inderal

PASS/FAIL

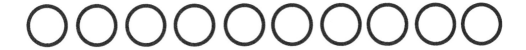

○○○○○○○○○○

GENERIC

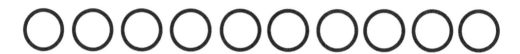

Hydralazine

Antihypertensive

PASS/FAIL

◯◯◯◯◯◯◯◯◯◯

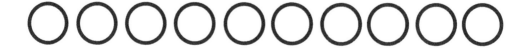

Propranolol

Antihypertensive

PASS/FAIL

◯◯◯◯◯◯◯◯◯◯

Brand

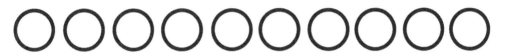

Verelan

PASS/FAIL

○○○○○○○○○○

Imitrex

PASS/FAIL

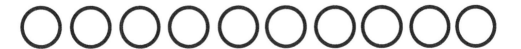

○○○○○○○○○○

GENERIC

Verapamil

Antihypertensive

PASS/FAIL

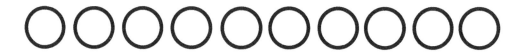

Sumatriptan

Antimigraine

PASS/FAIL

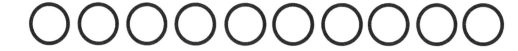

Brand

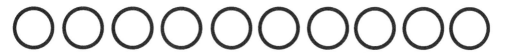

Seroquel

PASS/FAIL

○○○○○○○○○○

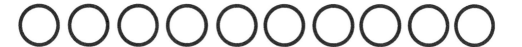

Abilify

PASS/FAIL

○○○○○○○○○○

GENERIC

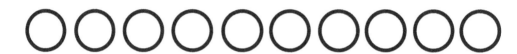

Quetiapine

Antipsychotic

PASS/FAIL

○○○○○○○○○○

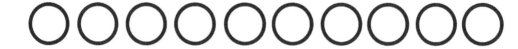

Aripiprazole

Antipsychotic

PASS/FAIL

○○○○○○○○○○

Brand

Zyprexa

PASS/FAIL

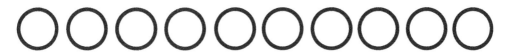

Risperdal

PASS/FAIL

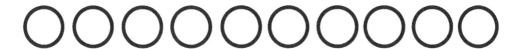

GENERIC

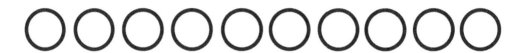

Olanzapine

Antipsychotic

PASS/FAIL

○○○○○○○○○○

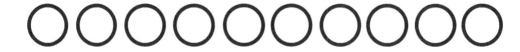

Risperidone

Antipsychotic

PASS/FAIL

○○○○○○○○○○

Brand

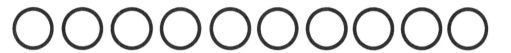

Latuda

PASS/FAIL

○○○○○○○○○○

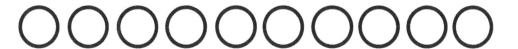

Rheumatrex

PASS/FAIL

○○○○○○○○○○

GENERIC

Lurasidone

Antipsychotic

PASS/FAIL

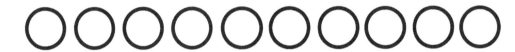

Methotrexate

Antirheumatic

PASS/FAIL

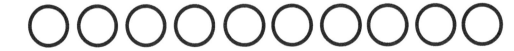

Brand

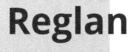

PASS/FAIL

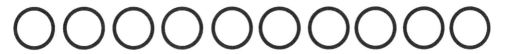

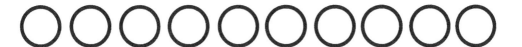

PASS/FAIL

GENERIC

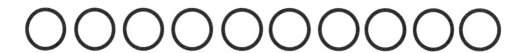

Metoclopramide

Antispasmodic

PASS/FAIL

○○○○○○○○○○

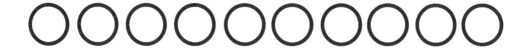

Dicyclomine

Antispasmodic

PASS/FAIL

○○○○○○○○○○

Brand

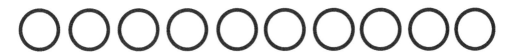

Tessalon

PASS/FAIL

○○○○○○○○○○

Valtrex

PASS/FAIL

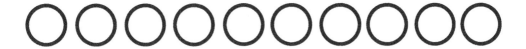

○○○○○○○○○○

GENERIC

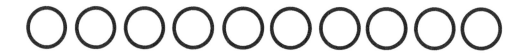

Benzonatate

Antitussive

○○○○○○○○○○

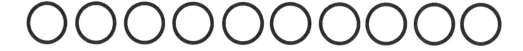

Valacyclovir

Antiviral

○○○○○○○○○○

Brand

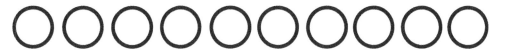

Zovirax

PASS/FAIL

◯◯◯◯◯◯◯◯◯◯

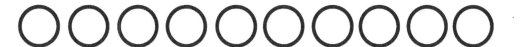

Tamiflu

PASS/FAIL

◯◯◯◯◯◯◯◯◯◯

GENERIC

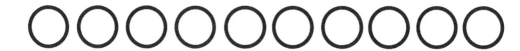

Acyclovir

Antiviral

PASS/FAIL

◯◯◯◯◯◯◯◯◯◯

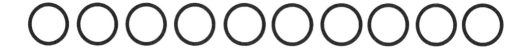

Oseltamivir

Antiviral

PASS/FAIL

◯◯◯◯◯◯◯◯◯◯

Brand

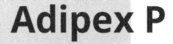

Adipex P

PASS/FAIL

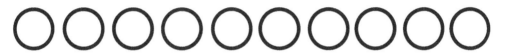

VESIcare

PASS/FAIL

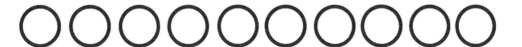

GENERIC

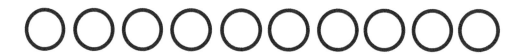

Phentermine

Appetite suppressant

PASS/FAIL

○○○○○○○○○○

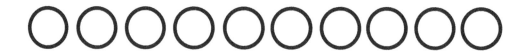

Solifenacin

Bladder relaxant

PASS/FAIL

○○○○○○○○○○

Brand

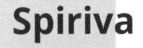

Spiriva

PASS/FAIL

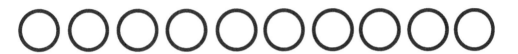

Daliresp

PASS/FAIL

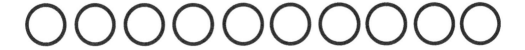

GENERIC

Tiotropium

C.O.P.D.

PASS/FAIL

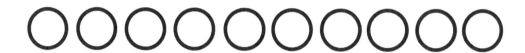

Roflumilast

C.O.P.D.

PASS/FAIL

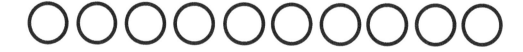

Brand

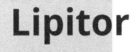

PASS/FAIL

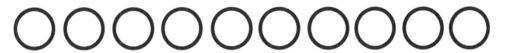

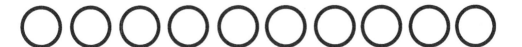

PASS/FAIL

OOOOOOOOOO

GENERIC

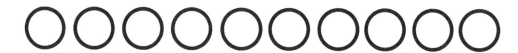

Atorvastatin

Cholesterol lowering

PASS/FAIL

○○○○○○○○○○

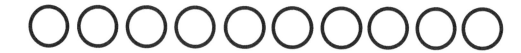

Simvastatin

Cholesterol lowering

PASS/FAIL

○○○○○○○○○○

Brand

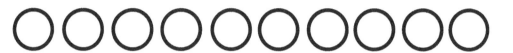

Crestor

PASS/FAIL

○○○○○○○○○○

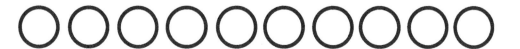

Mevacor

PASS/FAIL

○○○○○○○○○○

GENERIC

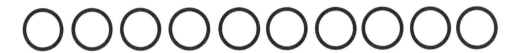

Rosuvastatin

Cholesterol lowering

PASS/FAIL

○○○○○○○○○○

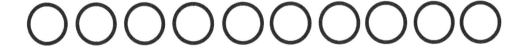

Lovastatin

Cholesterol lowering

PASS/FAIL

○○○○○○○○○○

Brand

Pravachol

PASS/FAIL

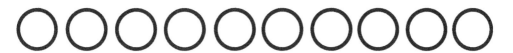

Zetia

PASS/FAIL

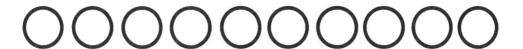

GENERIC

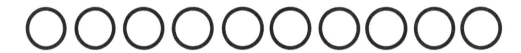

Pravastatin

Cholesterol lowering

PASS/FAIL

◯◯◯◯◯◯◯◯◯◯

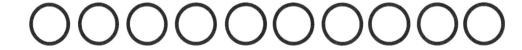

Ezetimibe

Cholesterol lowering

PASS/FAIL

◯◯◯◯◯◯◯◯◯◯

Brand

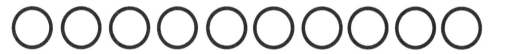

Niaspan

PASS/FAIL

OOOOOOOOOOO

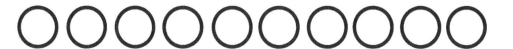

Lopid

PASS/FAIL

OOOOOOOOOO

GENERIC

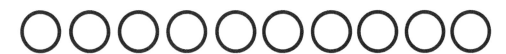

Niacin

Cholesterol lowering

PASS/FAIL

○○○○○○○○○○

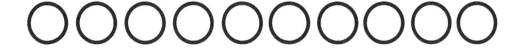

Gemfibrozil

Cholesterol lowering

PASS/FAIL

○○○○○○○○○○

Brand

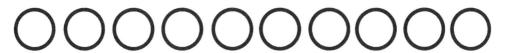

Juxtapid

PASS/FAIL

○○○○○○○○○○

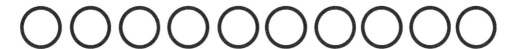

Vytorin

PASS/FAIL

○○○○○○○○○○

GENERIC

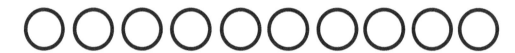

Lomitapide

Cholesterol lowering

PASS/FAIL

○○○○○○○○○○

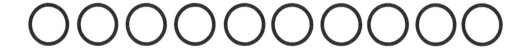

Ezetimibe / Simvastatin

Cholesterol lowering

PASS/FAIL

○○○○○○○○○○

Brand

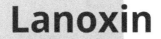

PASS/FAIL

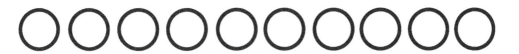

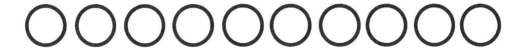

HCTZ

PASS/FAIL

GENERIC

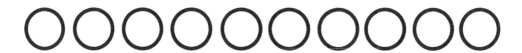

Digoxin

Congestive Heart Failure

PASS/FAIL

○○○○○○○○○○

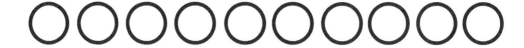

Hydrochlorothiazide

Diuretic

PASS/FAIL

○○○○○○○○○○

Brand

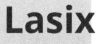

PASS/FAIL

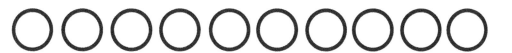

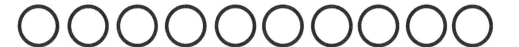

PASS/FAIL

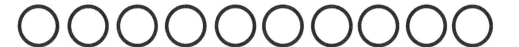

GENERIC

Furosemide

Diuretic

PASS/FAIL

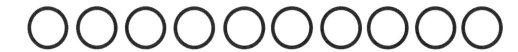

Triamterene/HCTZ

Diuretic

PASS/FAIL

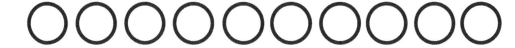

Brand

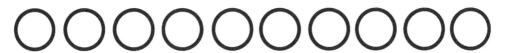

Aldactone

PASS/FAIL

○○○○○○○○○○

K-Tab

PASS/FAIL

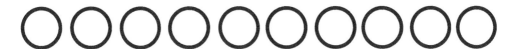

○○○○○○○○○○

GENERIC

Spironolactone

Diuretic

PASS/FAIL

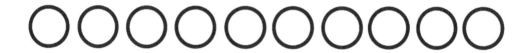

Potassium

Electrolyte

PASS/FAIL

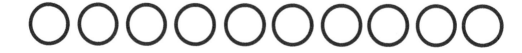

Brand

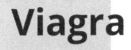

PASS/FAIL

OOOOOOOOOO

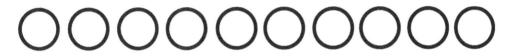

PASS/FAIL

OOOOOOOOOO

GENERIC

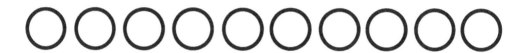

Sildenafil

Erectile dysfunction

PASS/FAIL

○○○○○○○○○○

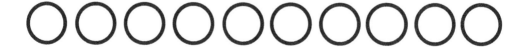

Vardenafil

Erectile dysfunction

PASS/FAIL

○○○○○○○○○○

Brand

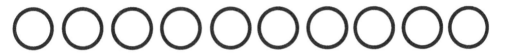

Cialis

PASS/FAIL

○○○○○○○○○○

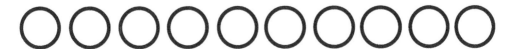

Robitussin

PASS/FAIL

○○○○○○○○○○

GENERIC

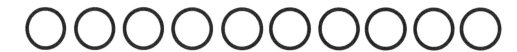

Tadalifil

Erectile dysfunction

PASS/FAIL

○○○○○○○○○○

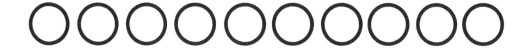

Guiafenesin

Expectorant

PASS/FAIL

○○○○○○○○○○

Brand

Synthroid

PASS/FAIL

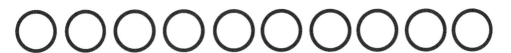

Premarin

PASS/FAIL

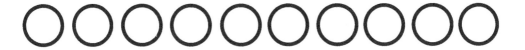

GENERIC

Levothyroxine

Hormone replacement

PASS/FAIL

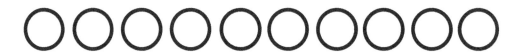

Estrogen

Hormone replacement

PASS/FAIL

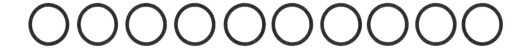

Brand

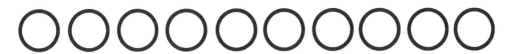

Armour Thyroid

PASS/FAIL

○ ○ ○ ○ ○ ○ ○ ○ ○ ○

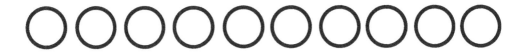

AndroGel

PASS/FAIL

○ ○ ○ ○ ○ ○ ○ ○ ○ ○

GENERIC

Thyroid

Hormone replacement

PASS/FAIL

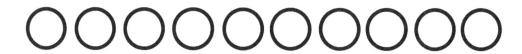

Testosterone

Hormone replacement

PASS/FAIL

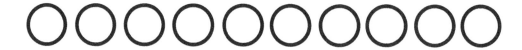

Brand

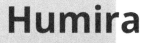

PASS/FAIL

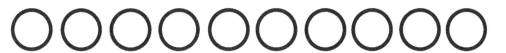

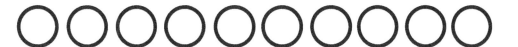

Detrol

PASS/FAIL

GENERIC

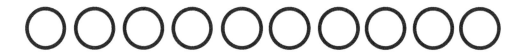

Adalimumab

Immunosuppressant

PASS/FAIL

○○○○○○○○○○

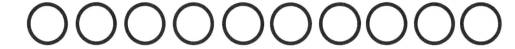

Tolterodine

Incontinence

PASS/FAIL

○○○○○○○○○○

Brand

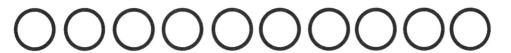

Ditropan

PASS/FAIL

○○○○○○○○○○

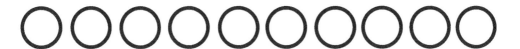

Flexeril

PASS/FAIL

○○○○○○○○○○

GENERIC

Oxybutynin

Incontinence

PASS/FAIL

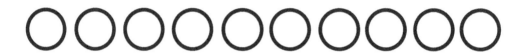

Cyclobenzaprine

Muscle Relaxer

PASS/FAIL

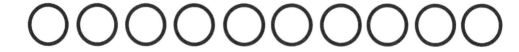

Brand

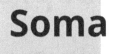

Soma

PASS/FAIL

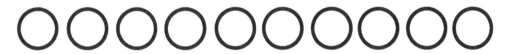

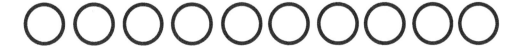

PASS/FAIL

GENERIC

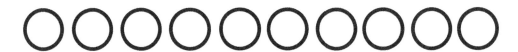

Carisoprodol

Muscle Relaxer

PASS/FAIL

○○○○○○○○○○

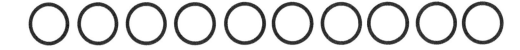

Methocarbamol

Muscle Relaxer

PASS/FAIL

○○○○○○○○○○

Brand

Zanaflex

PASS/FAIL

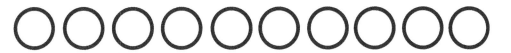

Suboxone

PASS/FAIL

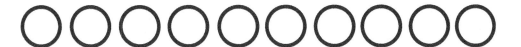

GENERIC

Tizanidine

Muscle Relaxer

PASS/FAIL

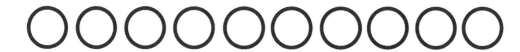

Buprenorphine / Naloxone

Opioid Addiction

PASS/FAIL

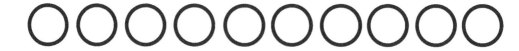

Brand

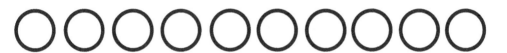

PASS/FAIL

○○○○○○○○○○

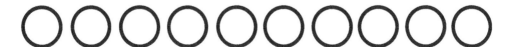

PASS/FAIL

○○○○○○○○○○

GENERIC

Methadone

Opioid addiction

PASS/FAIL

○○○○○○○○○○

Risedronate

Osteoporosis

PASS/FAIL

○○○○○○○○○○

Brand

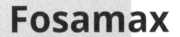

Fosamax

PASS/FAIL

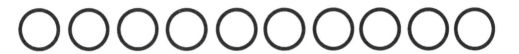

Evista

PASS/FAIL

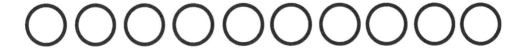

GENERIC

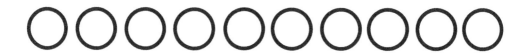

Alendronate

Osteoporosis

PASS/FAIL

○○○○○○○○○○

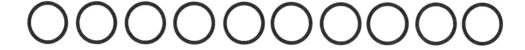

Raloxifene

Osteoporosis

PASS/FAIL

○○○○○○○○○○

Brand

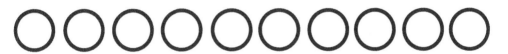

Zostavax

PASS/FAIL

○○○○○○○○○○

Ambien

PASS/FAIL

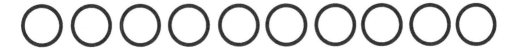

○○○○○○○○○○

GENERIC

Zoster Vaccine

Shingles Vaccine

PASS/FAIL

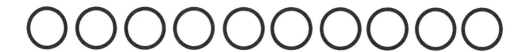

Zolpidem

Sleep aid

PASS/FAIL

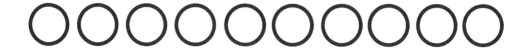

Brand

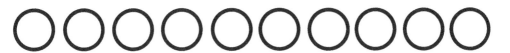

Lunesta

PASS/FAIL

○○○○○○○○○○

Restoril

PASS/FAIL

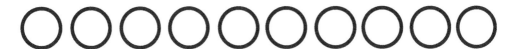

○○○○○○○○○○

GENERIC

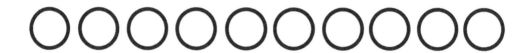

Eszopiclone

Sleep Aid

PASS/FAIL

○○○○○○○○○○

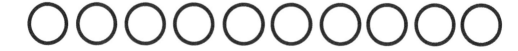

Temazepam

Class

PASS/FAIL

○○○○○○○○○○

Brand

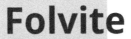

Folvite

PASS/FAIL

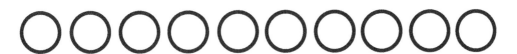

Caltrate

PASS/FAIL

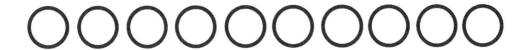

GENERIC

Folic Acid

Supplement

PASS/FAIL

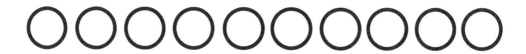

Vitamin D

Supplement

PASS/FAIL

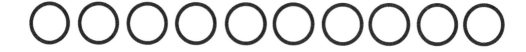

Brand

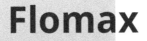

Flomax

PASS/FAIL

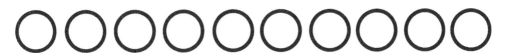

Cardura

PASS/FAIL

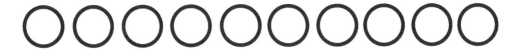

GENERIC

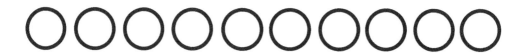

Tamsulosin

Urinary retention

PASS/FAIL

○○○○○○○○○○

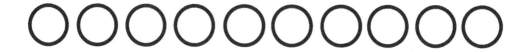

Doxazosin
Urinary retention / Antihypertensive

PASS/FAIL

○○○○○○○○○○

Brand

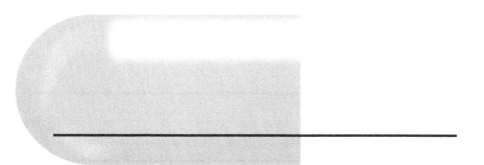

PASS/FAIL

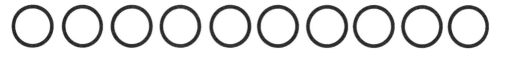

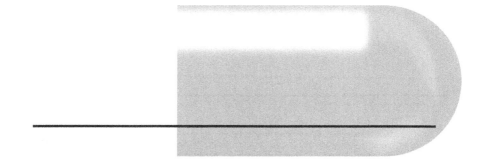

PASS/FAIL

GENERIC

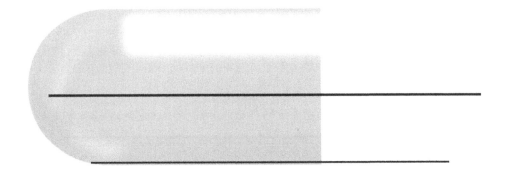

PASS/FAIL

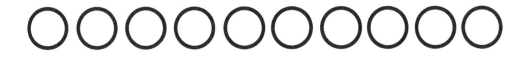

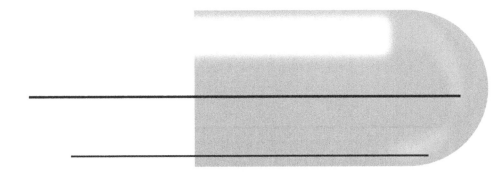

PASS/FAIL

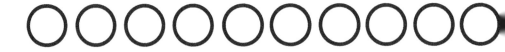

Brand

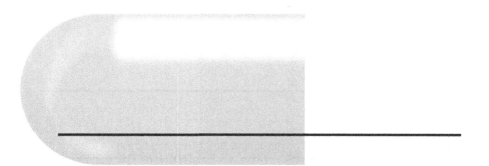

PASS/FAIL

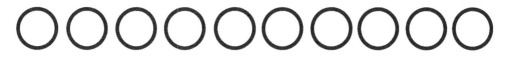

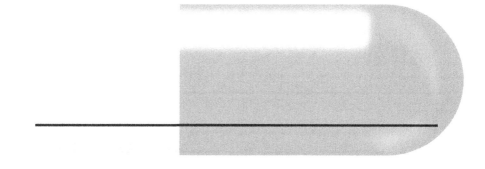

PASS/FAIL

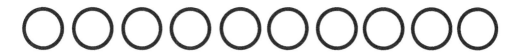

GENERIC

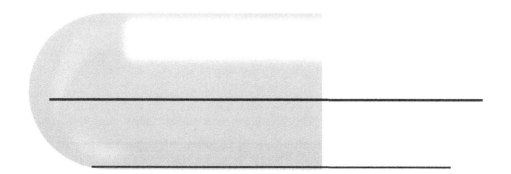

PASS/FAIL

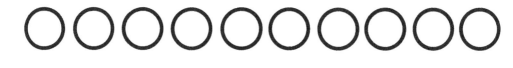

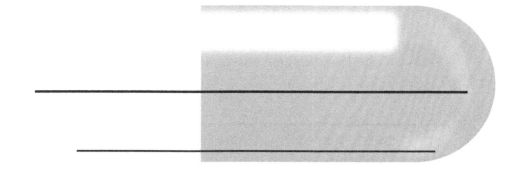

PASS/FAIL

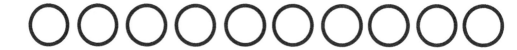

Notes

Notes

Notes

Made in United States
Orlando, FL
22 September 2024

51818567R00124